Table Of Contents

Chapter 1: Introduction to Polyamorous Marriages

Understanding Polyamory

Understanding polyamory involves delving into a relationship style that embraces love and intimacy with multiple partners, all while maintaining open communication and consent. At its core, polyamory challenges traditional notions of exclusivity in romantic relationships, offering a framework where love is not a finite resource but rather an expansive one. For couples considering or already engaged in polyamorous marriages, understanding the principles of polyamory can be the foundation for fostering healthy relationships. This section will explore the essential elements of polyamory, focusing on communication, emotional management, and the dynamics of family life.

Effective communication is paramount in polyamorous relationships. Unlike monogamous setups, where couples might rely on a singular partnership dynamic, polyamorous marriages require intentional dialogue about feelings, boundaries, and expectations. Couples must cultivate a practice of regular check-ins to discuss their emotional states, relationship dynamics, and any concerns that may arise. This proactive communication approach not only strengthens the bonds between partners but also helps in navigating the complexities that come with having multiple relationships. Utilizing tools such as active listening and nonviolent communication strategies can significantly enhance understanding and empathy among partners.

Jealousy and insecurity are common emotions that can surface in polyamorous relationships, often stemming from fears of inadequacy or fear of losing a partner's affection. Understanding these feelings is crucial for couples. Recognizing that jealousy can be a natural response, partners can work together to create a supportive environment where they can express these emotions without judgment. Strategies such as discussing triggers, establishing secure attachments, and reinforcing commitments can help mitigate feelings of jealousy. By approaching these emotions constructively, partners not only foster individual growth but also strengthen their collective bond.

Raising children in polyamorous families introduces unique dynamics and challenges that require thoughtful navigation. Parents must consider how to communicate their relationship structure to their children and address any questions or concerns they may have. Creating a stable and nurturing environment is essential, and this often involves discussing the importance of love, respect, and consent with children from an early age. It can also be beneficial to involve all adult partners in parenting decisions, ensuring a cohesive approach that reinforces the family unit. Support networks, including extended family and like-minded friends, can play a vital role in providing additional resources and emotional backing.

Personal growth and self-discovery are often highlighted as significant benefits of engaging in polyamorous relationships. For many individuals, the opportunity to explore connections outside their primary partnership can lead to profound insights about their desires, needs, and identity. Couples can support each other's journeys of self-discovery by encouraging exploration and self-reflection. This aspect of polyamory not only enriches individual lives but can also enhance the primary relationship as partners bring new perspectives and experiences to the table. Overall, understanding polyamory involves embracing its complexities while fostering a culture of open communication, mutual respect, and ongoing personal development within the marriage.

The Landscape of Modern Relationships

The landscape of modern relationships has evolved significantly over the past few decades, reflecting a broader acceptance of diverse relationship structures. Polyamorous marriages, characterized by consensual non-monogamy, are gaining visibility as couples seek alternatives to traditional monogamous frameworks. This shift invites a re-examination of communication strategies, emotional management, parenting approaches, and support systems, all of which are crucial for navigating the complexities of polyamorous dynamics. Understanding these elements is essential for couples looking to thrive in a polyamorous context.

Effective communication serves as the foundation for any relationship, and this is especially true in polyamorous marriages. Since partners may have multiple romantic connections, the need for clear, open dialogue becomes paramount. Couples must establish communication techniques that prioritize honesty and transparency while addressing the unique challenges of multiple relationships. Regular check-ins, active listening, and the use of "I" statements can foster an environment where all partners feel heard and valued. By honing these skills, couples can navigate the intricacies of their relationships with greater ease and understanding.

Jealousy and insecurity are common emotions that can arise in polyamorous relationships, often stemming from societal conditioning or personal insecurities. It is vital for couples to acknowledge these feelings and develop strategies to manage them constructively. Open discussions about triggers, boundaries, and individual needs can help partners address jealousy before it escalates. Practicing self-reflection and developing a strong sense of self-worth are equally important, as they empower individuals to recognize that their value is not diminished by the relationships of their partners. By fostering resilience and emotional intelligence, couples can create a strong foundation for navigating these challenges.

Parenting within a polyamorous framework presents unique dynamics and challenges that require thoughtful consideration. Couples need to engage in open discussions about their parenting philosophies, co-parenting strategies, and how to introduce children to the concept of polyamory in an age-appropriate manner. Building a cohesive family unit may involve establishing clear guidelines for interactions with multiple partners, ensuring that children feel secure and loved. Furthermore, creating a support network of like-minded families can provide additional resources and reassurance, allowing parents to share experiences and strategies that honor both their relationship choices and their children's well-being.

Support systems play a crucial role in the success of polyamorous marriages, offering couples a sense of community and belonging. Identifying and building these networks can be instrumental in providing emotional support, practical advice, and friendship. Couples may find value in connecting with local polyamory groups, online forums, or workshops focused on consensual non-monogamy. These platforms can help individuals navigate personal growth and self-discovery within their relationships. By engaging with others who share similar experiences, couples can foster resilience, learn from shared challenges, and celebrate their unique journeys, ultimately enhancing the richness of their polyamorous lives.

The Importance of Communication

Communication serves as the bedrock of any relationship, and this is especially true in polyamorous marriages where multiple emotional and romantic connections intertwine. The importance of communication cannot be overstated; it is the primary tool through which partners express their needs, boundaries, and feelings. In a polyamorous context, where partners may navigate complex dynamics and varying expectations, effective communication becomes crucial in fostering a sense of security and understanding. By mastering communication strategies, couples can create a strong foundation that allows each partner to feel heard, respected, and valued.

One of the primary challenges in polyamorous relationships is the potential for jealousy and insecurity. Open lines of communication are essential in addressing these feelings before they escalate into larger issues. Couples should cultivate an environment where they can openly discuss their emotions, including vulnerabilities and fears. This can involve regular check-ins, where partners take the time to share their feelings and experiences without fear of judgment. Such practices not only help in managing jealousy but also strengthen the emotional bonds among partners, as they learn to support one another through their insecurities.

In addition to emotional navigation, communication plays a vital role in the unique challenges of raising children in polyamorous families. Parents must discuss their parenting philosophies, values, and approaches to ensure that they present a united front to their children. This requires ongoing dialogue about how to address questions related to family structure and how to communicate with children about their diverse family dynamics. By sharing these conversations openly, parents can model effective communication for their children, encouraging them to express themselves and understand the nuances of their family environment.

Support systems are another critical aspect of polyamorous marriages, and effective communication can enhance the development of these networks. Couples should engage in conversations about their individual needs for support, whether through friendships, family connections, or community resources. By expressing their needs clearly, partners can help each other identify and cultivate supportive relationships with other individuals who understand the complexities of polyamory. This collaborative approach not only alleviates feelings of isolation but also reinforces the notion that no partner should face their challenges alone.

Ultimately, communication in polyamorous marriages also facilitates personal growth and self-discovery. As partners engage in open dialogues about their desires, aspirations, and boundaries, they create an atmosphere conducive to exploration. This process allows individuals to gain deeper insights into their own identities and relationship styles, promoting a sense of empowerment. By prioritizing communication, couples can foster an environment where personal growth is celebrated, and each partner feels free to embark on their journey of self-discovery, all while remaining committed to the collective health of their relationships.

Chapter 2: Communication Strategies in Polyamorous Marriages

The Foundation of Open Dialogue

The foundation of open dialogue in polyamorous marriages is essential for fostering healthy relationships among partners. Open dialogue goes beyond mere communication; it encompasses honesty, empathy, and a willingness to engage in difficult conversations. In polyamorous settings, where multiple emotional and romantic connections exist, maintaining clarity and understanding is crucial. This foundation allows couples to navigate the complexities of their relationships, ensuring that each partner feels heard and valued. Establishing this environment of open communication can significantly reduce misunderstandings and build trust, which is vital in any relationship but particularly in polyamorous dynamics.

Effective communication strategies are the bedrock of successful polyamorous marriages. Partners must cultivate a space where they can express their thoughts and feelings without fear of judgment or retribution. Techniques such as active listening, where one partner fully engages with what the other is saying, can help in understanding different perspectives. Additionally, regular check-ins can provide a structured opportunity for partners to discuss their feelings, desires, and any concerns that may arise. These practices not only strengthen the relationship but also empower individuals to articulate their needs, which is essential for maintaining balance among multiple partners.

Navigating feelings of jealousy and insecurity is another critical aspect of open dialogue. In polyamorous relationships, partners may experience envy or uncertainty about their place within the relationship structure. Open dialogue allows couples to address these feelings constructively rather than letting them fester. Sharing insecurities can lead to mutual reassurance and the development of coping strategies. For example, discussing specific triggers can help partners understand each other's emotional landscapes, providing a framework for support. By fostering this level of transparency, partners can work together to mitigate jealousy and build a stronger emotional connection.

Raising children in polyamorous families presents unique challenges that require open communication among all adults involved. It is essential for parents to discuss their values and parenting philosophies openly to ensure consistency in how children are raised. Open dialogue can help create a cohesive family environment where children feel secure and loved by all parental figures. Moreover, discussing potential scenarios related to parenting—such as how to handle questions from children about their family structure—can prepare partners for these conversations, promoting a united front and reducing confusion for the children.

Finally, the personal growth and self-discovery that often occur in polyamorous marriages can be greatly enhanced by maintaining a foundation of open dialogue. As partners engage in conversations about their experiences, feelings, and aspirations, they create opportunities for each other's growth. This shared journey encourages individuals to explore their identities and desires within the context of their relationships. By fostering an environment where personal exploration is celebrated and supported, couples can strengthen their bonds and enrich their lives. Ultimately, the foundation of open dialogue not only facilitates effective communication but also nurtures the growth and evolution of each partner, leading to a more fulfilling polyamorous marriage.

Active Listening Techniques

Active listening is a fundamental communication technique that can enhance understanding and connection among partners in polyamorous marriages. In an environment where multiple emotional dynamics and relationships coexist, the ability to listen actively becomes even more critical. Active listening involves not only hearing the words spoken but also understanding the underlying feelings and intentions. This technique fosters a deeper connection between partners, allowing them to express their needs and concerns without fear of judgment. In polyamorous arrangements, where partners may experience unique challenges such as jealousy and insecurity, honing active listening skills can significantly improve the quality of communication and emotional safety.

One effective active listening technique is to use reflective listening. This involves paraphrasing what the speaker has said to confirm understanding. For example, if one partner expresses feelings of jealousy regarding another relationship, the listener can respond with, "It sounds like you're feeling insecure about my time with [name]. Is that right?" Reflective listening not only validates the speaker's emotions but also encourages them to elaborate further. This technique creates a safe space for open dialogue, allowing partners to explore their feelings and concerns in a constructive manner. It is particularly beneficial for navigating the complexities of polyamorous relationships, where emotions can be intense and multifaceted.

Another vital component of active listening is maintaining eye contact and appropriate body language. Non-verbal cues convey attentiveness and empathy, making it clear to the speaker that their feelings are being acknowledged. Partners should aim to eliminate distractions during conversations, such as silencing phones or turning off the television, to demonstrate commitment to the discussion. By focusing entirely on the speaker, partners can better understand the nuances of what is being communicated, which is essential when addressing sensitive topics related to jealousy, insecurity, or even parenting decisions within a polyamorous family.

In addition to reflective listening and non-verbal cues, asking open-ended questions can significantly enhance active listening. These questions encourage deeper exploration of thoughts and feelings. Instead of asking, "Are you upset about this?" a partner might ask, "What specifically makes you feel uncomfortable about our arrangement?" This approach invites more substantial dialogue and gives the other partner the opportunity to share their perspective comprehensively. Such conversations can reveal underlying issues that may not have been addressed, ultimately promoting personal growth and self-discovery within the relationship.

Lastly, it is important for partners to practice patience and avoid interrupting when someone is speaking. Interruptions can create feelings of resentment and discourage open communication. Allowing each partner to fully express themselves before responding not only demonstrates respect but also enhances the overall quality of the conversation. In polyamorous marriages, where partners may face unique challenges and dynamics, prioritizing active listening can help cultivate a supportive environment. This approach not only strengthens individual relationships but also fosters a healthy collective partnership, enabling couples to navigate the complexities of polyamory with clarity and compassion.

The Role of Non-Verbal Communication

The role of non-verbal communication in polyamorous marriages is pivotal for fostering understanding and deepening connections among partners. While verbal communication lays the groundwork for sharing thoughts and feelings, non-verbal cues often convey emotions and intentions that words alone cannot express. In polyamorous relationships, where multiple dynamics and emotional landscapes coexist, being attuned to non-verbal signals can help partners navigate complex interactions, mitigate misunderstandings, and enhance emotional intimacy. This subchapter will explore how non-verbal communication functions within polyamorous marriages, emphasizing its importance in strengthening relationships.

One of the most significant aspects of non-verbal communication is body language, which encompasses gestures, posture, and facial expressions. In a polyamorous setting, where partners may have varying levels of comfort and familiarity, being sensitive to these signals can help identify unspoken feelings. For instance, a partner's crossed arms or lack of eye contact might indicate discomfort or insecurity, prompting a conversation about underlying issues. By recognizing and addressing these non-verbal cues, couples can create a safe space for open dialogue, enabling them to confront jealousy or insecurity before they escalate into larger conflicts.

Touch is another crucial element of non-verbal communication that can reinforce emotional bonds in polyamorous marriages. Different partners may have varying preferences for physical affection, making it essential to understand and respect these boundaries. A comforting touch, a reassuring hug, or even a gentle squeeze of the hand can convey support and affirmation, fostering a sense of belonging and acceptance. In the context of raising children within a polyamorous family, modeling healthy non-verbal communication can also set a positive example for younger generations, demonstrating the importance of empathy and understanding in interpersonal relationships.

Facial expressions serve as powerful indicators of emotional states and can significantly influence how partners engage with one another. In polyamorous relationships, where partners may experience a range of emotions simultaneously, being aware of each other's expressions can facilitate better emotional regulation. For instance, a partner's smile might signal contentment and joy, while a furrowed brow could indicate confusion or concern. By paying attention to these subtle cues, couples can develop a deeper emotional literacy, enabling them to support each other more effectively through life's challenges and transitions.

Lastly, the role of non-verbal communication extends beyond individual interactions to encompass the broader dynamics of support systems within polyamorous marriages. Couples can benefit from engaging with their community, attending workshops, or participating in support groups where non-verbal communication plays a role in building rapport and trust. Shared experiences can create a sense of unity and mutual understanding among partners, allowing them to navigate the complexities of polyamory together. By honing their non-verbal communication skills, couples can enrich their relationships, mitigate feelings of jealousy and insecurity, and foster personal growth, ultimately leading to a more harmonious and fulfilling polyamorous marriage.

Setting Boundaries and Expectations

Setting boundaries and expectations is a crucial aspect of maintaining healthy dynamics in polyamorous marriages. As couples navigate the complexities of multiple relationships, clear communication about personal limits and relationship expectations becomes essential. Establishing boundaries helps partners create a safe emotional space where they can express their needs and feelings without fear of judgment or misunderstanding. These boundaries can encompass a wide range of areas, including emotional, physical, and time commitments, and should be revisited regularly as relationships evolve.

When discussing boundaries, it is vital for couples to engage in open and honest conversations. This involves not only articulating personal needs but also actively listening to each partner's perspective. Effective communication strategies, such as using "I" statements and avoiding accusatory language, can foster a more productive dialogue. For example, instead of saying, "You always ignore my needs," a partner might express, "I feel neglected when we don't spend quality time together." This shift in language can reduce defensiveness and encourage a more empathetic exchange. The goal is to ensure that each partner feels heard and validated, which strengthens the foundation of trust necessary for polyamorous relationships.

Jealousy and insecurity can often arise in polyamorous settings, making it crucial to establish boundaries that address these feelings. Couples should proactively discuss what triggers jealousy and how to manage those emotions constructively. This may include setting parameters around time spent with other partners, sharing information about new relationships, or agreeing on specific times for dedicated couple time. By acknowledging these feelings and creating a plan to address them, partners can reduce tension and foster a more supportive environment. Regular check-ins can also help partners reassess their comfort levels and make adjustments to their boundaries as needed.

Raising children in polyamorous families adds another layer of complexity to boundary setting. Couples must navigate not only their personal relationships but also the implications for their children. It is essential to establish clear expectations regarding family dynamics, discipline, and the involvement of additional partners in parenting roles. Open discussions about how to explain polyamory to children, as well as how to handle questions or concerns they may have, will help in creating a cohesive family environment. By setting these boundaries, couples can ensure that their children grow up in a loving and understanding atmosphere, where they feel secure in their family structure.

Building a support system is another important aspect of establishing boundaries and expectations within polyamorous marriages. Couples should identify friends, family members, or community groups that are supportive of their relationship structure and can provide emotional backing when challenges arise. This network can offer guidance on navigating difficult conversations, dealing with jealousy, or managing parenting responsibilities. Furthermore, engaging with other polyamorous families can provide valuable insights and strategies that enhance personal growth and self-discovery. By creating a supportive environment, couples not only fortify their own relationships but also contribute to the broader polyamorous community, fostering shared understanding and growth.

Regular Check-Ins

Regular check-ins are a critical component of effective communication in polyamorous marriages. These structured conversations offer couples the opportunity to address any issues, share feelings, and reinforce their commitments to each other and their other partners. By establishing a routine for these discussions, couples can create a safe space to explore thoughts and emotions that may otherwise remain unspoken. This proactive approach not only helps to mitigate misunderstandings but also fosters a deeper emotional intimacy among partners.

When navigating the complexities of polyamorous relationships, feelings of jealousy and insecurity can emerge. Regular check-ins provide a platform for partners to express these feelings openly. During these discussions, couples can validate each other's emotions, clarify intentions, and collaboratively devise strategies to address any concerns. This practice reinforces trust and allows partners to work through their vulnerabilities together, ultimately transforming potentially divisive feelings into opportunities for growth and understanding.

Raising children in a polyamorous family brings unique dynamics that require careful consideration and communication. Regular check-ins can serve as a framework for discussing parenting philosophies, boundaries, and the emotional well-being of all family members involved. By engaging in these conversations, parents can align their approaches to child-rearing, ensuring that children receive consistent messages about love, acceptance, and the diverse forms relationships can take. Furthermore, these discussions can help in addressing any anxieties related to how polyamory may impact the children's lives, allowing parents to be proactive in creating a supportive environment.

Support systems are vital for polyamorous couples, and regular check-ins can also extend to include discussions about external networks. These conversations can help partners identify the resources they need, whether that be friends, family, or community groups, to navigate the unique challenges of their relationships. By articulating their needs and seeking support together, couples can strengthen their bond and enhance their resilience against external pressures. This proactive approach ensures that partners feel less isolated and more empowered in their journey, reinforcing their commitment to one another.

Finally, regular check-ins facilitate personal growth and self-discovery within polyamorous marriages. These discussions encourage individuals to reflect on their own needs, desires, and aspirations, promoting a culture of self-exploration. When partners share their personal journeys during check-ins, they not only enhance their own understanding but also contribute to each other's growth. This mutual support enhances the relationship, allowing both partners to thrive as individuals while remaining deeply connected. In this way, regular check-ins become a powerful tool for fostering a healthy, evolving polyamorous marriage where communication is prioritized, and personal development is celebrated.

Chapter 3: Navigating Jealousy and Insecurity

Understanding Jealousy in Polyamory

Understanding jealousy in polyamory is a crucial aspect for couples navigating the complexities of multiple romantic relationships. Jealousy, often seen as a negative emotion, can emerge in polyamorous settings just as it does in monogamous relationships. However, the dynamics are different; in polyamory, partners must confront not only their feelings but also the beliefs and assumptions that underpin those emotions. This subchapter explores the roots of jealousy, how it manifests in polyamorous marriages, and effective strategies for addressing it while fostering open communication.

At its core, jealousy often stems from insecurities and fears of inadequacy. In a polyamorous context, these feelings can be amplified by the presence of additional partners. Couples may grapple with the fear of being replaced or the worry that their partner's affection is being divided. Understanding these underlying triggers is essential to addressing jealousy constructively. By recognizing that jealousy often reflects personal insecurities rather than the actions of others, couples can begin to dismantle the harmful narratives that fuel these emotions.

Open communication is key in managing jealousy. Partners should create safe spaces to discuss their feelings without judgment or defensiveness. Regular check-ins can help partners express their concerns and vulnerabilities before they escalate into significant issues. Utilizing "I" statements can be particularly effective; for example, saying "I feel insecure when you spend time with your other partner" instead of "You make me feel insecure" fosters a more collaborative dialogue. By encouraging honest discussions about feelings, couples can strengthen their emotional bonds and build a deeper understanding of each other's needs.

In addition to communication, developing personal strategies to cope with jealousy is beneficial. Mindfulness practices, such as meditation or journaling, can help individuals process their emotions healthily. Setting boundaries that honor each partner's comfort levels is also crucial. These boundaries might include time allocations for different partners or specific agreements about how to share experiences and resources. Such strategies empower individuals to take ownership of their feelings, reducing the likelihood of jealousy disrupting the overall harmony of the relationship.

Lastly, building a robust support system is integral to navigating jealousy in polyamorous marriages. Engaging with other polyamorous couples or support groups can provide valuable perspectives and strategies for managing feelings of jealousy. These networks can also offer reassurance that such emotions are common and manageable. By fostering connections with others who understand the unique challenges of polyamorous dynamics, couples can find solidarity and encouragement in their journey towards personal growth and relationship fulfillment. In this way, jealousy can transform from a source of conflict into an opportunity for deeper understanding and connection within polyamorous families.

Identifying Triggers and Patterns

Identifying triggers and patterns is a crucial step for couples navigating the complexities of polyamorous marriages. Recognizing the emotional responses that can arise in these relationships is essential for fostering healthy communication and promoting mutual understanding. By pinpointing specific triggers—situations or interactions that provoke strong emotional reactions—partners can better anticipate and address challenges before they escalate. This awareness not only enhances communication but also creates an environment where each individual feels safe to express their feelings without fear of judgment or misunderstanding.

One common trigger in polyamorous settings is the feeling of jealousy, which can arise from various sources such as perceived neglect, unequal attention from partners, or comparisons with others. Identifying the root cause of jealousy is vital for managing it effectively. Couples can benefit from discussing their feelings openly, exploring what specifically makes them feel insecure or threatened. By engaging in these conversations, partners can develop strategies to mitigate jealousy, such as establishing clear boundaries and affirming each other's importance in the relationship. Through this process, couples can create a supportive dialogue that helps to normalize these feelings rather than suppress them.

Recognizing patterns in behavior is equally important in understanding the dynamics of polyamorous relationships. Patterns may manifest in recurring conflicts, communication breakdowns, or emotional responses to specific situations. Couples should take time to reflect on past experiences, identifying moments when emotions ran high and the underlying factors involved. By examining these patterns, partners can gain insights into their triggers and work collaboratively to adjust their responses. This proactive approach not only helps in resolving conflicts but also fosters a deeper emotional connection as both partners learn to navigate their vulnerabilities together.

When raising children in a polyamorous family, identifying triggers and patterns also plays a significant role. Children can be sensitive to the emotional climate of their household, and parents must be mindful of how their dynamics affect their well-being. Open discussions about family structure and emotional health can help children feel secure and understood. Parents should also recognize patterns in their parenting styles and communication with children, ensuring that all caregivers are on the same page. This consistency reinforces a sense of stability and support, allowing children to thrive in a polyamorous environment.

Building a robust support system is another critical factor in identifying triggers and patterns. Couples in polyamorous marriages often benefit from connecting with like-minded individuals who understand the unique challenges they face. Support groups, online forums, or community events can provide valuable insights and strategies for managing emotions and navigating complex dynamics. By sharing experiences with others, couples can learn to identify common triggers and patterns, equipping them with tools to enhance their communication and strengthen their relationships. Ultimately, this collective wisdom can lead to personal growth and a deeper understanding of oneself and one's partners within the context of a polyamorous marriage.

Techniques for Managing Jealousy

Managing jealousy in polyamorous marriages is essential for fostering a healthy, supportive, and communicative environment. Jealousy can arise from various sources, including fear of losing a partner, insecurity about self-worth, and concerns over unequal attention. Recognizing that these feelings are natural can be the first step toward addressing them constructively. Couples can implement specific techniques to manage jealousy, transforming it from a destructive force into an opportunity for growth, understanding, and deeper connection.

One effective technique for managing jealousy is open communication. Couples should establish a safe space where they can express their feelings without judgment. This involves actively listening to each other and validating emotions, even if they seem irrational. Practicing nonviolent communication can help in articulating needs and concerns without placing blame. For example, instead of saying, "You are spending too much time with your other partner," one might express, "I feel anxious when I perceive a shift in our time together." This approach encourages empathy and understanding, allowing partners to navigate their emotions collectively.

Another important strategy is self-reflection. Partners should take time to explore the root causes of their jealousy. Is it stemming from past experiences, insecurities, or unmet needs? Journaling or engaging in self-discovery activities can provide insights into personal triggers and motivations. By understanding these underlying factors, individuals can communicate their needs more effectively and seek reassurance from their partners. This process not only reduces jealousy but also promotes personal growth, leading to a stronger sense of self within the relationship.

Setting clear boundaries is also crucial in managing jealousy. Couples should discuss and agree on what is comfortable and acceptable for both partners in the relationship. This may include guidelines around time spent with other partners, emotional availability, or physical intimacy. Having these boundaries in place creates a sense of security, as partners know what to expect from one another. Regularly revisiting and adjusting these boundaries as the relationship evolves can further alleviate feelings of jealousy, as it reinforces the commitment to each other and the relationship's health.

Lastly, cultivating a support system can significantly aid in managing jealousy. Engaging with other polyamorous couples or individuals can provide a sense of community and shared experience. Support groups, whether online or in-person, can offer valuable perspectives and coping strategies. Additionally, seeking professional guidance from therapists who specialize in polyamory can facilitate deeper discussions around jealousy and insecurity. Establishing a robust support network not only helps couples navigate their feelings but also fosters a sense of belonging and understanding within the broader polyamorous community. By employing these techniques, couples can transform jealousy into a catalyst for growth and connection, ultimately strengthening their polyamorous marriage.

Building Trust Among Partners

Building trust among partners in polyamorous marriages is a foundational aspect that can significantly enhance the quality of relationships and promote a healthy, supportive environment. Trust is not merely a passive state; it requires active cultivation through consistent communication, transparency, and mutual respect. In a polyamorous context, where multiple emotional and romantic connections exist, the need for trust becomes even more pronounced. Partners must engage in open dialogues about their feelings, boundaries, and expectations to create a solid base of trust that can withstand the unique challenges of polyamory.

Effective communication strategies play a critical role in fostering trust. Partners should prioritize regular check-ins to discuss their emotional states, relationship dynamics, and any concerns that may arise. These conversations can include sharing feelings of jealousy or insecurity, which are often heightened in polyamorous arrangements. By openly addressing these feelings rather than suppressing them, partners can work together to reassure one another and reaffirm their commitment. Incorporating tools such as reflective listening—where one partner paraphrases what the other has said—can enhance understanding and empathy, ensuring that both partners feel heard and valued.

Navigating jealousy and insecurity is another significant challenge in polyamorous marriages. It is essential for partners to acknowledge and validate these emotions rather than dismiss them. Creating a safe space for vulnerability allows partners to express their fears and insecurities without fear of judgment. Techniques such as expressing gratitude for each other and highlighting the unique qualities each partner brings can help mitigate feelings of competition. Through this process, partners not only build trust but also strengthen their emotional bonds by reaffirming their commitment to one another amidst the complexities of their relationships.

Raising children in polyamorous families introduces additional dimensions to the trust-building process. It's crucial for partners to present a united front and establish consistent parenting practices, which can be more complex with multiple caregivers involved. Open communication about parenting styles, expectations, and the roles each partner will play is vital. This collaborative approach not only builds trust among the adult partners but also provides children with a stable and supportive environment. When children see their parents communicating effectively and working together harmoniously, they learn the importance of trust and cooperation in relationships.

Lastly, building support systems for polyamorous couples can significantly enhance trust among partners. Engaging with community resources, attending workshops, or joining support groups can provide valuable insights and practical strategies for navigating the unique challenges of polyamorous living. These networks can serve as a sounding board for partners, offering perspectives that reinforce trust and understanding. By surrounding themselves with supportive individuals who share similar experiences, partners can feel more secure in their choices and better equipped to handle the complexities of their relationships. Ultimately, the journey of building trust is ongoing, requiring continuous effort, communication, and commitment from all partners involved.

Emotional Regulation Strategies

Emotional regulation is a critical component in maintaining healthy communication and relationships within polyamorous marriages. In a dynamic where multiple partners are involved, each partner brings their own emotions, insecurities, and experiences into the mix. This complexity can lead to heightened feelings of jealousy, anxiety, and confusion, making it essential for couples to develop strategies that help them navigate these emotional landscapes effectively. By understanding and implementing emotional regulation techniques, partners can foster a more harmonious and fulfilling connection, enhancing their overall experience in a polyamorous setting.

One effective strategy for emotional regulation is the practice of mindfulness. Mindfulness encourages individuals to become aware of their thoughts and feelings without judgment. Couples can benefit from dedicating time to reflect on their emotions, allowing them to identify triggers that may lead to jealousy or insecurity. By recognizing these feelings in the moment, partners can communicate openly about their experiences rather than allowing unresolved emotions to fester. Engaging in mindfulness exercises, such as meditation or breathing techniques, can help partners stay grounded and present, providing a foundation for more constructive conversations.

Another useful approach involves establishing clear communication channels. Regular check-ins, where partners openly discuss their feelings and needs, can create an atmosphere of trust and support. These conversations should focus on expressing emotions without blame or criticism, fostering an environment where individuals feel safe to share their vulnerabilities. Couples can use "I" statements to articulate their feelings, such as "I feel anxious when I think about you spending time with someone else," which can reduce defensiveness and promote understanding. By prioritizing open dialogue, partners can collaboratively work through their emotions, reinforcing their bond and commitment to one another.

Additionally, it is essential for couples to cultivate self-compassion and empathy. Recognizing that jealousy and insecurity are natural human emotions can help partners approach these feelings with kindness rather than self-judgment. By practicing self-compassion, individuals can better understand their emotional responses and learn to manage them effectively. Empathy plays a crucial role in this process, as partners who actively seek to understand each other's perspectives can mitigate feelings of isolation and fear. This mutual support can strengthen the relationship, providing a solid foundation for personal growth and emotional exploration.

Finally, building a robust support system is vital for emotional regulation in polyamorous marriages. Connecting with other polyamorous couples or joining community groups can provide partners with valuable insights and coping strategies. Having a network of individuals who understand the unique challenges of polyamory can alleviate feelings of loneliness and provide reassurance. Couples can also seek professional support, such as therapy or counseling, to navigate complex emotions and develop tailored strategies for emotional regulation. By investing in both personal and communal resources, partners can enhance their emotional resilience, creating a more supportive and nurturing environment within their polyamorous marriage.

24

Chapter 4: Raising Children in Polyamorous Families

The Unique Dynamics of Polyamorous Parenting

The dynamics of polyamorous parenting introduce a rich tapestry of relationships that can significantly enhance the family experience when navigated thoughtfully. In polyamorous families, children have the unique opportunity to engage with multiple parental figures, each bringing distinct perspectives, values, and skills to their upbringing. This diversity can foster a nurturing environment filled with varied support systems, allowing children to learn from a range of experiences and viewpoints. However, the complexity of these dynamics necessitates clear communication among all adults involved to ensure that the children receive consistent messages and support.

Effective communication strategies are paramount in managing the unique challenges of polyamorous parenting. Each partner must prioritize open discussions about roles, responsibilities, and expectations in the parenting process. Regular family meetings can be an excellent way to facilitate dialogue among all caregivers, allowing them to express concerns, celebrate successes, and make collective decisions regarding the children's upbringing. This practice not only reinforces a sense of unity among the adults but also models healthy communication skills for the children, teaching them the importance of expressing their thoughts and feelings openly.

Jealousy and insecurity can pose significant challenges in polyamorous relationships, particularly when children are involved. Parents may grapple with feelings of inadequacy or fear of not being the primary influence in their child's life. To address these emotions, it is essential for partners to engage in self-reflection and communicate their feelings openly. Establishing reassurances about each person's role and significance in the child's life can mitigate these feelings. Additionally, creating opportunities for one-on-one time with each child can reinforce individual bonds, alleviating concerns about competition for affection and attention.

Raising children in a polyamorous context also necessitates the establishment of robust support systems. In many cases, polyamorous families may face societal stigma or misunderstanding, which can create additional stress. Building a network of like-minded families or supportive friends who understand the polyamorous lifestyle can provide both emotional and practical support. This network can serve as a resource for sharing experiences, offering advice, and fostering a sense of community. Additionally, being part of such a network can validate the family structure and provide children with peers who share similar backgrounds, helping them navigate their own social interactions.

Lastly, polyamorous parenting can serve as a catalyst for personal growth and self-discovery among the adults involved. The complexities of managing multiple relationships compel individuals to confront their insecurities and develop greater emotional intelligence. This process can lead to enriched personal development, as parents learn to balance their own needs with those of their family. Embracing the challenges of polyamorous parenting can inspire a deeper understanding of love, commitment, and resilience, ultimately enhancing the quality of relationships within the family unit. As parents grow together, they not only enrich their own lives but also instill valuable lessons in their children about love, acceptance, and the importance of communication.

Communication with Children About Polyamory

Communication about polyamory with children is a nuanced and sensitive topic that requires careful consideration and a thoughtful approach. As couples navigate their polyamorous relationships, it is crucial to recognize that children are often curious and perceptive. They may notice the dynamics of their parents' relationships and have questions or feelings that need to be addressed. Open and age-appropriate communication can foster understanding and create a supportive environment where children feel safe exploring their own feelings about love and relationships.

One effective strategy for discussing polyamory with children is to tailor the conversation to their developmental stage. Younger children may not need intricate details but can benefit from simple explanations about love and relationships. For instance, parents might describe polyamory as having multiple loving relationships, emphasizing that love is not a finite resource. This framing helps children understand that their parents' love for them remains unchanged, regardless of other relationships. As children grow older and their cognitive abilities develop, parents can introduce more complex concepts surrounding consent, boundaries, and emotional dynamics, allowing for an enriching dialogue that respects their evolving understanding.

Addressing potential feelings of jealousy or insecurity in children is equally important. Children may worry that they will lose their parents' attention or love due to the presence of additional partners. To alleviate these concerns, couples should actively reassure their children of their commitment and affection. Regular family activities and one-on-one time can reinforce the bond between parents and children, illustrating that love can be abundant rather than divided. Open discussions about feelings of jealousy can also empower children to express their emotions, helping them to develop healthy coping mechanisms and emotional intelligence as they grow.

Building a support system is essential for polyamorous couples when it comes to parenting. Engaging with others who share similar experiences can provide valuable insights and resources for navigating the complexities of raising children in a polyamorous household. Support groups, online communities, or local meet-ups can serve as platforms for sharing strategies, challenges, and successes. These networks can also offer emotional support, helping parents to feel less isolated and more confident in their parenting approach. By fostering connections with other polyamorous families, couples can learn from one another and reinforce the idea that diverse family structures can thrive.

Lastly, the journey of parenting within a polyamorous framework can serve as a catalyst for personal growth and self-discovery. As parents navigate the intricacies of their relationships alongside their parenting responsibilities, they often confront their own beliefs and values. This process can lead to greater self-awareness and emotional maturity. Couples can use these experiences to model healthy relationships for their children, showcasing the importance of communication, respect, and integrity. By openly discussing their own learnings and challenges, parents can inspire their children to embrace their individuality and encourage them to explore their own paths in love and relationships.

Co-Parenting Strategies in Polyamorous Marriages

Co-parenting in polyamorous marriages presents unique challenges and opportunities that require intentional communication and collaboration among all involved parties. At the core of successful co-parenting lies a strong foundation of open dialogue. Couples must prioritize regular discussions about parenting styles, values, and expectations. Establishing a shared vision for raising children can help mitigate misunderstandings and ensure that all parents are aligned in their approach. This alignment not only fosters a stable environment for the children but also strengthens the relationships among the adults involved, creating a unified front that the children can trust.

Managing feelings of jealousy and insecurity is paramount when navigating co-parenting in a polyamorous context. The presence of multiple partners can sometimes trigger emotions that complicate parenting dynamics. It is essential for partners to engage in proactive emotional check-ins where they can express their feelings without fear of judgment. This practice not only cultivates empathy but also allows partners to address insecurities in a constructive manner. By acknowledging these feelings and discussing them openly, couples can work together to find solutions that benefit both their relationships and their children.

Raising children in polyamorous families involves navigating differing opinions on parenting methods. To facilitate harmony, it is beneficial to establish clear roles and responsibilities among all parents. This clarity prevents overlap and confusion, allowing each parent to contribute their strengths to the family unit. Regular family meetings can serve as a platform for discussing parenting strategies, resolving conflicts, and celebrating successes. By involving children in age-appropriate discussions about their family structure, parents can promote understanding and acceptance, helping children to feel secure in their unique family dynamics.

Support systems are crucial for polyamorous couples, especially when it comes to co-parenting. Building a network of friends, family, and fellow polyamorous families can provide essential resources and emotional support. Engaging with community groups focused on polyamory can offer valuable insights and strategies from others who have navigated similar challenges. Additionally, these connections can create a sense of belonging and validation for both adults and children, reinforcing the idea that their family structure is a legitimate and healthy choice.

Personal growth and self-discovery are integral to the journey of co-parenting in polyamorous marriages. The challenges that arise can serve as opportunities for individuals to explore their values, beliefs, and parenting philosophies. Embracing the fluid nature of polyamorous relationships allows partners to learn from one another, adapt to changing circumstances, and foster resilience. By approaching co-parenting as a shared adventure, couples can not only enhance their relationships but also model positive coping strategies for their children, ultimately contributing to a nurturing and dynamic family environment.

Addressing Societal Stigmas

Addressing societal stigmas is a crucial element in fostering healthy communication within polyamorous marriages. Stigmas, often rooted in traditional views of monogamy, can create barriers that undermine the emotional security and trust necessary for effective communication. Couples navigating polyamorous dynamics frequently encounter judgment from family, friends, and society at large, which can amplify feelings of isolation and insecurity. Recognizing these stigmas is the first step toward dismantling their impact and creating a supportive environment for open dialogue.

One effective communication strategy for addressing societal stigmas is the practice of open and honest discussions with all partners involved. This includes not only sharing feelings about external perceptions but also exploring how these views affect individual experiences within the relationship. Couples can benefit from regular check-ins to discuss any external influences, ensuring that everyone feels heard and validated. This proactive approach helps to alleviate misunderstandings and promotes a unified front against societal pressures, reinforcing the bond among partners.

Navigating feelings of jealousy and insecurity is another critical aspect influenced by societal stigmas. When external opinions suggest that polyamory is inherently flawed or less valid than monogamous relationships, individuals may internalize these beliefs, leading to self-doubt and relational tensions. To counteract this, couples should cultivate an environment of reassurance, where partners can express vulnerabilities without fear of judgment. By acknowledging and addressing jealousy as a natural emotion rather than a flaw, couples can develop strategies to manage these feelings constructively. This may involve creating agreements or boundaries that address specific insecurities, fostering a sense of safety and understanding.

When raising children in polyamorous families, societal stigmas can pose unique challenges. Parents must navigate how to communicate their family structure to their children and address any questions or concerns that may arise from external sources. Open communication with children about relationships can normalize polyamory and foster acceptance from a young age. It is essential for parents to create a narrative that emphasizes love and commitment, regardless of the number of partners involved. Engaging children in discussions about love, respect, and diversity can help dismantle societal biases and instill a sense of confidence in their family structure.

Finally, building support systems is vital for polyamorous couples facing societal stigmas. Connecting with other polyamorous families or joining community groups can provide a sense of belonging and validation. These networks offer opportunities for sharing experiences and strategies for dealing with external challenges, reinforcing the idea that polyamory is a legitimate and fulfilling lifestyle. Additionally, seeking out resources such as workshops or counseling, specifically designed for polyamorous relationships, can equip couples with tools to address stigmas more effectively. By fostering a supportive community, couples can strengthen their relationships and cultivate personal growth, transforming societal challenges into opportunities for deeper connection and understanding.

Creating a Supportive Environment for Children

Creating a supportive environment for children in polyamorous families requires intentionality and communication. As couples navigate the complexities of their relationships, it is crucial to prioritize the emotional and psychological well-being of their children. This involves establishing a foundation where children feel secure, loved, and understood, regardless of the various dynamics present in their family structure. To achieve this, couples must engage in open dialogues not only with each other but also with their children, fostering an atmosphere where feelings and thoughts can be expressed without fear of judgment.

Effective communication strategies play a pivotal role in cultivating a supportive environment. Parents should aim to create regular opportunities for family discussions, where each member can share their experiences and emotions. This practice not only strengthens familial bonds but also teaches children the importance of expressing their feelings. When parents model healthy communication, children are more likely to adopt these skills themselves, preparing them for future relationships and social interactions. Furthermore, using age-appropriate language and concepts can help children understand the dynamics of their family structure, ensuring they feel included and informed.

Navigating feelings of jealousy and insecurity is another critical aspect of creating a nurturing environment. Children can sense emotional tensions, and if not addressed, these feelings can manifest as anxiety or behavioral issues. Parents must openly discuss their own feelings and challenges within the polyamorous framework, providing reassurance to their children that love and commitment are not diminished by the presence of multiple relationships. Creating a narrative that emphasizes love's abundance rather than scarcity can help children develop a healthier perspective on relationships, teaching them that it is possible to love many while still maintaining deep bonds with each individual.

Raising children in a polyamorous setting also underscores the importance of robust support systems. Building a network of like-minded families, friends, and community members who understand and respect the polyamorous lifestyle can provide invaluable resources for parents. These connections can offer emotional support, shared experiences, and practical advice for navigating parenting challenges unique to polyamorous families. Furthermore, involving children in social activities with other polyamorous families can help normalize their experiences, fostering a sense of belonging and understanding of their family structure.

Lastly, personal growth and self-discovery within polyamorous marriages can significantly enhance the supportive environment for children. When parents engage in their own self-exploration and growth, they become more attuned to their emotional needs and those of their children. This self-awareness fosters a nurturing atmosphere where children are encouraged to pursue their interests and develop their identities. By demonstrating the value of personal growth and healthy relationships, parents can inspire their children to embrace their individuality and navigate their own relationships with confidence and compassion. In this way, the family unit not only thrives but also becomes a model for future generations of open-hearted communication and connection.

Chapter 5: Support Systems for Polyamorous Couples

Identifying Personal Support Networks

Identifying personal support networks is a crucial aspect of thriving in polyamorous marriages. These networks serve as essential resources, providing emotional, social, and practical support that can help couples navigate the complexities of their relationships. Understanding who these supporters are and how they contribute to individual and collective well-being is imperative. This subchapter will explore the various dimensions of personal support networks, including their importance, the types of support available, and strategies for building and maintaining these connections.

The foundation of a robust personal support network often begins with open communication among partners about their needs and feelings. In polyamorous marriages, where multiple relationships come into play, it is vital to articulate what individuals require from their partners and their extended network. This includes discussing feelings of jealousy, insecurity, and the challenges of parenting in a non-traditional family structure. Establishing a shared understanding of each partner's emotional landscape can facilitate deeper connections not only within the marriage but also with external supporters, such as friends, family, and fellow polyamorous individuals.

Support networks can take various forms, ranging from close friends and family members to community groups and online forums. Each of these sources can provide different types of assistance, whether it be emotional validation, practical advice, or shared experiences. Friends who understand polyamory can offer insights that resonate with the unique dynamics of a polyamorous marriage, while family members may provide a sense of stability and belonging, albeit sometimes with more traditional views. Identifying which individuals or groups align with your values and needs can help you create a diverse and reliable support system.

Building and maintaining a personal support network requires intentionality and effort. Start by identifying individuals who are empathetic and open-minded, as these qualities are essential for providing constructive support. Regularly check in with these individuals, whether through informal chats, scheduled gatherings, or social media interactions. Additionally, consider joining local or online polyamorous communities that offer resources, workshops, and social events. Engaging with others who share similar experiences can help validate your feelings and provide practical strategies for managing the complexities of polyamorous relationships.

Ultimately, personal support networks play a vital role in fostering personal growth and self-discovery within polyamorous marriages. They not only provide emotional support but also encourage individuals to explore their identities and desires without fear of judgment. A well-rounded network can inspire couples to confront challenges together and celebrate their successes, reinforcing the notion that polyamory can be a source of strength and resilience. By identifying and nurturing these support systems, couples can enhance their communication, navigate jealousy and insecurity, and cultivate a fulfilling family life, ultimately leading to a richer and more harmonious polyamorous existence.

Building Community Connections

Building community connections is essential for polyamorous couples seeking to navigate the complexities of their relationships. Unlike traditional monogamous partnerships, polyamorous marriages thrive on open communication, mutual support, and shared experiences among multiple partners. Establishing a community can provide a vital network of understanding and encouragement, allowing couples to feel less isolated in their unique relationship dynamics. This community can take various forms, from local meetups and online forums to more structured support groups, all of which foster shared experiences and collective wisdom.

For couples engaged in polyamorous relationships, effective communication strategies are paramount. Building community connections offers a platform for couples to share their experiences, challenges, and triumphs. Regular discussions with peers can help partners develop new communication techniques that may be beneficial in their own relationships. Engaging with others who face similar challenges allows couples to learn from each other and refine their approaches to communication, ultimately enhancing the overall quality of their relationships. This collaborative environment reinforces the idea that no couple is alone in their journey, and collective problem-solving can yield innovative solutions.

Navigating feelings of jealousy and insecurity is another critical aspect of polyamorous marriages, and community connections can play a pivotal role in addressing these emotional challenges. When couples share their feelings with others who understand the intricacies of polyamory, they can gain insights into managing jealousy and insecurity more effectively. Support from a community can validate a partner's feelings while also providing alternative perspectives that may help diffuse intense emotions. In this way, community connections become a valuable resource for emotional support, allowing couples to confront and process their feelings in a safe and constructive environment.

For those raising children in polyamorous families, building connections within a community can help navigate the unique dynamics and challenges of parenting. Engaging with other polyamorous families can provide practical advice, emotional support, and shared resources that address the complexities of parenting in a non-traditional family structure. Whether it's discussing co-parenting strategies or sharing experiences about introducing children to the concept of polyamory, community connections can foster a sense of solidarity among parents. This collective knowledge can help ease the burden of parenting decisions, ensuring that children grow up in an environment that embraces diversity and open-mindedness.

Finally, the journey of personal growth and self-discovery is enhanced through community connections. Polyamory often encourages individuals to explore their identities and desires within the context of their marriages. Engaging with a supportive community provides opportunities for self-reflection and growth, as members share their own journeys of self-discovery. Whether it's through workshops, discussion groups, or informal gatherings, the exchange of ideas and experiences can inspire personal development. By cultivating these connections, polyamorous couples not only strengthen their relationships but also foster a culture of growth and exploration that benefits all members involved.

The Role of Support Groups

Support groups play a pivotal role in the lives of couples navigating the complexities of polyamorous marriages. These groups provide a safe space for individuals to share their experiences, challenges, and triumphs, fostering an environment of understanding and acceptance. Within these supportive networks, couples can engage in open dialogues about the unique aspects of their relationships, including communication strategies, jealousy management, and the dynamics of raising children in a polyamorous context. By participating in support groups, partners not only find camaraderie but also learn invaluable skills that can enhance their relationships.

Effective communication is the cornerstone of any successful polyamorous marriage, and support groups often serve as a training ground for honing these skills. Within these settings, couples can practice active listening, express their needs, and articulate their feelings without fear of judgment. Through role-playing scenarios and guided discussions, partners can explore various communication techniques that can help mitigate misunderstandings and foster deeper connections. This collaborative learning environment empowers individuals to refine their communication styles, ensuring that every voice is heard and valued, which is essential in maintaining harmony in multifaceted relationships.

Jealousy and insecurity are common emotions that can arise in polyamorous marriages, and support groups offer a platform to address these feelings openly. Members can share their personal experiences with jealousy and learn from one another's coping strategies. This collective wisdom can help couples identify triggers and develop proactive measures to manage these emotions. By discussing jealousy in a supportive environment, partners can dismantle the stigma surrounding these feelings, realizing they are not alone in their struggles. Such discussions can lead to practical solutions, fostering trust and transparency, which are vital for the health of any polyamorous relationship.

Raising children in polyamorous families presents its own set of challenges, and support groups can provide essential guidance and resources. Parents can connect with others who share similar experiences, exchanging tips on navigating societal perceptions, co-parenting dynamics, and maintaining open lines of communication with children. These groups can also facilitate discussions about how to instill values of love, acceptance, and honesty in children, preparing them to understand and appreciate diverse family structures. By engaging with other polyamorous families, couples can gain insights into best practices for parenting within their unique framework, ultimately benefiting their children's emotional and social development.

Beyond the immediate benefits of communication and parenting strategies, support groups also play a crucial role in personal growth and self-discovery. Engaging with others in similar situations allows individuals to reflect on their own journeys and aspirations within the context of polyamory. Participants often find inspiration in the stories of others, motivating them to explore their interests and desires more fully. This environment of shared vulnerability fosters self-exploration, encouraging individuals to embrace their authentic selves while remaining committed to their partners. In essence, support groups not only bolster the strength of polyamorous marriages but also contribute to the individual growth of each partner, enriching the relational tapestry of the family as a whole.

Utilizing Professional Help

Utilizing professional help can be a game-changer for couples navigating the complexities of polyamorous marriages. Many partners find that the challenges they face—whether related to communication, jealousy, parenting, or personal growth—can sometimes feel overwhelming. Engaging with professionals such as therapists or counselors who specialize in polyamory can provide invaluable insights and strategies. These experts are equipped to facilitate discussions that can enhance understanding, promote emotional safety, and help partners articulate their needs and concerns more effectively.

Effective communication strategies are crucial in any relationship, but they take on added complexity in polyamorous setups. Professionals can guide couples in establishing clear communication norms, such as regular check-ins and open discussions about feelings and boundaries. They can also introduce tools like "I" statements to express personal experiences without placing blame, fostering a more constructive dialogue. By working with a professional, couples can learn how to navigate difficult conversations about their relationships, ensuring that each partner feels heard and validated.

Jealousy and insecurity are common challenges in polyamorous marriages. When multiple emotional bonds are involved, it's natural for individuals to experience feelings of inadequacy or fear of loss. A trained therapist can help couples unpack these feelings, offering strategies to recognize triggers and address them collaboratively. Techniques such as cognitive-behavioral therapy can be employed to reframe negative thought patterns, while mindfulness practices can equip partners to manage their emotional responses more effectively. Through professional guidance, couples can develop a healthier perspective on jealousy, transforming it from a potential relationship strain into an opportunity for deeper connection and understanding.

Raising children in a polyamorous family presents its own unique dynamics and challenges. Professionals specializing in family therapy can assist couples in creating a cohesive parenting strategy that incorporates the values of all partners involved. They can help navigate discussions with children about family structure and ensure that conversations are age-appropriate and sensitive. Additionally, professionals can support parents in establishing boundaries and agreements that respect each partner's role and involvement, ultimately fostering a nurturing environment for children to thrive in a polyamorous context.

Finally, personal growth and self-discovery are integral components of polyamorous marriages. Engaging with a professional can facilitate individual exploration within the relationship framework, allowing partners to pursue their interests while maintaining a strong connection with one another. Therapists can encourage self-reflection and assist partners in identifying personal goals that align with their shared life, promoting a culture of growth and support. Ultimately, utilizing professional help can empower couples to navigate the intricacies of their polyamorous marriage, transforming challenges into opportunities for deeper connection and fulfillment.

Encouraging Friendships and Family Support

Encouraging friendships and family support is essential in fostering a resilient and harmonious environment within polyamorous marriages. In these relationships, the dynamics can become intricate due to the multiple connections involved, making it crucial to cultivate a network of understanding friends and family. Building this support system not only enhances communication but also helps mitigate feelings of jealousy and insecurity, which can arise in polyamorous settings. By openly discussing the nature of polyamory with loved ones, couples can create a foundation of trust and acceptance that benefits everyone involved.

One effective strategy for encouraging support from friends and family is to engage in open dialogues about the principles and values that underpin polyamory. Couples should consider hosting informal gatherings or discussions where they can share their experiences, answer questions, and address any misconceptions. This not only demystifies polyamory but also allows friends and family to voice their concerns or curiosities in a safe environment. By fostering these conversations, couples can help their loved ones understand that polyamory is built on love, trust, and communication, rather than competition or betrayal.

Another important aspect is to actively involve friends and family in the polyamorous journey. This can include inviting them to social events, family gatherings, or even celebrations that acknowledge the unique structure of the relationship. Such inclusivity reinforces the notion that polyamory is not just about romantic entanglements but also about building a broader community of support. When family and friends feel included, they are more likely to provide emotional backing and understanding, helping to alleviate feelings of isolation that some polyamorous individuals may experience.

Navigating the complexities of raising children in a polyamorous environment also benefits significantly from strong friendships and family support. It is vital for children to witness healthy relationships and understand that love can take many forms. By involving supportive family members and friends, parents can create a nurturing environment where children feel secure and accepted. This extended network can offer additional resources for parenting, providing a broader range of perspectives and experiences that enrich the family dynamic.

Finally, personal growth and self-discovery are often amplified through the support of friends and family in polyamorous marriages. When individuals feel backed by their loved ones, they are encouraged to explore their identities and desires more freely. This sense of security not only enhances individual well-being but also strengthens the relationship as a whole. By prioritizing the cultivation of friendships and family support, polyamorous couples can create a thriving ecosystem that nurtures communication, fosters understanding, and promotes emotional resilience. ultimately leading to a more fulfilling and harmonious partnership.

Chapter 6: Personal Growth and Self-Discovery in Polyamorous Marriages

The Intersection of Polyamory and Personal Development

The intersection of polyamory and personal development is a rich and transformative space for couples navigating the complexities of non-monogamous relationships. In polyamorous marriages, partners often find themselves embarking on a journey of self-discovery that is deeply intertwined with their emotional and relational experiences. This dynamic encourages individuals to explore their identities, desires, and boundaries in ways that can lead to profound personal growth. As couples engage in open communication and share their feelings, they create a fertile ground for understanding not only their partners but also themselves.

Effective communication strategies are essential in this context, as they can help partners articulate their needs and navigate the challenges of polyamory. Couples are encouraged to practice active listening, ensuring that each partner feels heard and valued. This involves not only expressing thoughts and emotions openly but also being receptive to feedback and differing perspectives. By fostering an environment of trust and transparency, couples can better manage the complexities of their relationships, ultimately enhancing their personal development as they learn to express vulnerability and authenticity.

Jealousy and insecurity are common challenges in polyamorous arrangements, often serving as catalysts for personal growth. As partners confront these feelings, they are presented with an opportunity to delve into their insecurities and understand their origins. This process can be transformative, allowing individuals to develop greater emotional resilience and self-awareness. By employing strategies to manage these emotions—such as open dialogues about feelings, setting clear boundaries, and engaging in self-reflection—couples can turn potentially destructive feelings into opportunities for growth and deeper connection.

Another critical aspect of personal development in polyamorous families is the experience of raising children within this framework. Parenting in a polyamorous setting introduces unique dynamics that require parents to model effective communication and emotional intelligence for their children. Discussing polyamory openly and honestly can provide children with a broader understanding of love and relationships, fostering acceptance and compassion. As parents navigate this terrain, they also engage in their own growth, learning how to balance their needs with those of their children while instilling values of honesty, respect, and open-mindedness.

Building a robust support system is vital for couples in polyamorous marriages, as it can significantly enhance their personal development journey. Engaging with like-minded individuals or communities can provide a sense of belonging and validation, reducing feelings of isolation that may arise. Support systems can include friends, family, or even professional networks that understand the nuances of polyamory. By connecting with others who share similar experiences and values, couples can gain insights, share strategies, and receive encouragement, ultimately contributing to their individual and collective growth within the context of their relationships.

Encouraging Individual Interests and Hobbies

Encouraging individual interests and hobbies is essential in polyamorous marriages, as it fosters personal growth and enriches the relationship dynamic. In a polyamorous context, where multiple connections can exist simultaneously, it is crucial for each partner to maintain their identities outside the primary relationship. Encouraging each other to pursue individual interests not only cultivates self-discovery but also enhances communication among partners, as they bring new experiences and insights into their interactions. This practice can help mitigate feelings of jealousy and insecurity, as partners become more secure in their individuality and less reliant on the relationship for their sense of self-worth.

When partners actively support each other's hobbies and interests, they create a safe space for individual expression. This environment nurtures self-exploration, allowing each person to delve into activities that resonate with their passions. Whether it's painting, hiking, or learning a new language, these pursuits can lead to personal fulfillment and a greater sense of autonomy. By prioritizing personal interests, couples can develop a deeper understanding of each other's unique desires and motivations, which ultimately strengthens their bond. This shared understanding fosters open communication, as partners feel more comfortable discussing their individual experiences and the ways these experiences shape their relationship.

Managing feelings of jealousy and insecurity is another critical aspect of encouraging individual interests. When partners are engaged in fulfilling activities outside the relationship, they can feel more confident in the love and commitment they share. This confidence can diminish the fear of losing their partner's affection to someone else. As individuals gain satisfaction from their personal pursuits, they become less likely to project their insecurities onto their partners. Instead, they can celebrate each other's successes and interests, creating an atmosphere of support rather than competition. This shift can lead to healthier dynamics where jealousy is acknowledged but not allowed to dictate the terms of the relationship.

For families with children, encouraging individual interests can also positively impact parenting dynamics within a polyamorous framework. Parents who engage in their hobbies are often more fulfilled and balanced, which can translate into a more nurturing environment for their children. When kids observe their parents pursuing passions, they learn the importance of self-care and personal growth, instilling these values in the next generation. Additionally, parents can share their interests with their children, fostering family bonding while also allowing for individual exploration. This balance can lead to a more cohesive family unit, where each member feels valued for their unique contributions.

Building a robust support system is essential for polyamorous couples navigating individual interests. Encouraging partners to connect with friends or communities that share similar passions can provide additional emotional and social support. These networks can offer encouragement and validation outside the primary relationship, reducing the burden on partners to fulfill every emotional need. By participating in activities with others who share their interests, partners can cultivate their identities and return to their relationship with renewed energy and perspectives. Ultimately, by fostering individual interests and hobbies, polyamorous couples can create a thriving environment that promotes personal growth, effective communication, and a deeper connection between partners.

Self-Reflection Practices

Self-reflection practices are essential for couples navigating the complexities of polyamorous marriages. These practices encourage partners to engage in deep personal introspection, fostering an environment where individual needs and emotions can be understood and articulated. By dedicating time to self-reflection, partners can identify their own feelings of jealousy or insecurity, recognize patterns in their behavior, and gain clarity on their desires and boundaries. This process not only enhances personal growth but also strengthens communication between partners, allowing for healthier interactions and a more supportive relationship dynamic.

One effective self-reflection practice is journaling, which allows individuals to explore their thoughts and emotions in a structured manner. Couples can dedicate time each week to write about their experiences, feelings, and any challenges they face within their polyamorous framework. This practice can help clarify emotions that may seem overwhelming in the heat of the moment. For instance, when feelings of jealousy arise, journaling can provide a safe space to dissect those emotions and understand their root causes. By sharing insights from their journals with one another, partners can engage in open discussions about their vulnerabilities, ultimately fostering a deeper connection and mutual understanding.

Another valuable practice is mindfulness meditation, which can help individuals become more attuned to their emotional states and reactions. Through mindfulness, partners can learn to observe their thoughts without judgment, creating space to reflect on their feelings in real-time. This practice is particularly beneficial when navigating difficult conversations or confronting insecurities within the relationship. By cultivating a mindfulness practice, couples can approach discussions about jealousy or boundary-setting with greater calmness and clarity, reducing the likelihood of misunderstandings and emotional outbursts.

Setting aside regular check-in sessions is also crucial for self-reflection in polyamorous marriages. These dedicated times allow partners to discuss their feelings, experiences, and any changes in their emotional landscape. During these check-ins, couples can explore how their self-reflection practices have informed their perspectives and decisions. This structured communication fosters accountability, as partners can support each other's growth while addressing any emerging issues. By creating a safe space for these discussions, couples can reinforce their commitment to open dialogue, ultimately reinforcing their emotional bond.

Finally, engaging in self-reflection within a supportive community can enhance the process significantly. Connecting with other polyamorous couples or individuals who share similar experiences can provide valuable insights and encouragement. Participating in workshops or support groups focused on personal growth and communication can introduce new self-reflection techniques and broaden perspectives. Sharing experiences and strategies with others can illuminate paths for growth that may not have been previously considered, enriching the individual journeys of each partner and fortifying the collective strength of the marriage. By embracing self-reflection practices, couples can navigate the complexities of polyamory with greater ease, fostering a nurturing environment for both personal and relational development.

Navigating Identity Within a Polyamorous Framework

Navigating identity within a polyamorous framework requires a conscious effort to articulate and explore one's sense of self in relation to multiple partners. In traditional monogamous relationships, identity often becomes intertwined with that of one's partner, leading to a shared sense of self. However, in polyamorous marriages, each partner must engage in self-reflection to understand their unique identities while also considering how these identities interact with the identities of others. This exploration can foster a richer understanding of oneself and one's relationship dynamics, promoting a stronger foundation for communication and connection.

Effective communication strategies are crucial in navigating identity within a polyamorous context. Partners should prioritize open dialogue about their individual identities, desires, and boundaries. Regular check-ins can help ensure that all partners feel seen and heard, allowing for adjustments and growth in the relationship. Practicing active listening and expressing vulnerability can deepen connections and foster a safe space for each person to explore their identity without fear of judgment or misunderstanding. By creating an environment where partners can express their evolving selves, couples can strengthen their bonds while honoring individual growth.

Jealousy and insecurity can surface when identities are challenged or when partners feel threatened by the presence of others. It is essential for polyamorous couples to develop strategies to manage these emotions. Acknowledging feelings of jealousy as natural and discussing them openly can lead to greater understanding and reassurance among partners. Establishing individual and collective coping mechanisms—such as sharing affirmations of love and commitment—can help mitigate these feelings. By tackling jealousy head-on and reframing it as an opportunity for growth, couples can navigate these challenges while maintaining a supportive environment for each other's identities.

Raising children within a polyamorous family introduces additional complexities regarding identity. Children may have questions about their family structure, and it is vital for parents to communicate openly about their relationships and the diverse identities within the family. This transparency helps children understand and embrace their family dynamics, fostering acceptance and resilience. Parents can also model healthy communication and emotional management, teaching their children valuable skills that will serve them in their own relationships. By prioritizing discussions about identity and relationships, polyamorous families can create a nurturing environment that celebrates diversity and individuality.

Building supportive networks is another essential aspect of navigating identity in polyamorous marriages. Couples can benefit greatly from connecting with other polyamorous families or communities, where shared experiences can provide valuable insights and foster a sense of belonging. These support systems can offer encouragement and resources for managing identity challenges and celebrating personal growth. By engaging with others who understand the unique dynamics of polyamory, couples can enhance their communication skills, learn new strategies for emotional management, and ultimately create a more fulfilling and authentic relationship framework.

Celebrating Growth and Change

Celebrating growth and change in polyamorous marriages is a vital aspect of nurturing both individual and collective relationships. As couples engage in non-monogamous dynamics, they often encounter various challenges and opportunities for personal and relational development. This subchapter explores the transformative journey that partners embark on, emphasizing the importance of recognizing and celebrating milestones, both big and small. By fostering an environment that values growth, couples can create a deeper emotional connection and a more fulfilling partnership.

Effective communication strategies play a crucial role in navigating the complexities of polyamorous relationships. Open dialogues about feelings, expectations, and boundaries can help couples understand each other's perspectives and experiences. When partners celebrate their growth together, they reinforce the idea that change is a natural part of any relationship. Acknowledging each other's achievements—whether it be managing jealousy, successfully integrating a new partner, or expanding emotional resilience—can foster a sense of unity and support. This shared acknowledgment not only strengthens the bond between partners but also encourages a culture of transparency that is essential for healthy communication.

Jealousy and insecurity are common emotions that arise in polyamorous marriages. Celebrating the growth in managing these feelings is vital for both individual and relational health. Couples can benefit from recognizing their progress in addressing jealousy, whether through open discussions or by developing coping strategies. When partners openly celebrate moments of vulnerability and transformation, they create a safe space for expressing insecurities without fear of judgment. This practice not only diminishes the weight of jealousy but also reinforces the commitment to growth, showing that partners are willing to navigate challenges together and emerge stronger.

Raising children in a polyamorous family presents unique dynamics that require intentional communication and collaboration. As parents celebrate their growth as individuals and as a collective unit, they model healthy relationship behaviors for their children. This can include discussions about love, acceptance, and the importance of community, which are essential values in polyamorous families. Celebrating the adaptation and successes in parenting—such as creating a supportive environment for children to understand diverse family structures—can empower parents and reaffirm their commitment to fostering an inclusive atmosphere. The act of celebrating these milestones can also strengthen the parental bond, enhancing the overall family dynamic.

Support systems are indispensable in polyamorous marriages, as they provide couples with the necessary tools to navigate their unique challenges and celebrate their journey. Engaging with like-minded individuals, whether through support groups or community events, allows couples to share experiences, strategies, and insights. Celebrating growth within these networks helps couples realize they are not alone in their journey. By highlighting successes—such as improved communication, successful integration of partners, or enhanced emotional awareness—couples can inspire one another and cultivate a sense of belonging. Ultimately, recognizing and celebrating growth and change within polyamorous marriages fosters resilience, deepens connections, and enhances the overall experience of love and partnership.

Chapter 7: Conclusion

Reflecting on the Journey

Reflecting on the journey of navigating a polyamorous marriage offers couples a unique opportunity to assess their communication strategies, confront feelings of jealousy and insecurity, and understand the complexities of raising children within a non-traditional family structure. This reflection is not merely an exercise in retrospection; it serves as a critical tool for personal growth and the strengthening of relationships. As partners progress through their experiences, they can identify what has worked well and what areas might still need attention or improvement. This subchapter aims to encapsulate the multifaceted aspects of this journey, encouraging couples to embrace their experiences as a pathway to deeper connection and understanding.

Effective communication is foundational in any relationship, but it takes on heightened importance in polyamorous marriages. Partners are encouraged to engage in open dialogues about their feelings, desires, and boundaries. Reflecting on past conversations can reveal patterns that either foster connection or create division. Couples may find that regular check-ins, where they discuss their emotional states and relationship dynamics, can help maintain clarity and prevent misunderstandings. By acknowledging the growth that happens through these discussions, partners can cultivate a healthier communication framework that not only addresses immediate concerns but also promotes long-term relational health.

Jealousy and insecurity are common challenges in polyamorous relationships, and reflecting on how these feelings have been managed over time can provide valuable insights. Couples might consider instances where jealousy arose and evaluate the responses that followed. Did they communicate openly about their feelings, or did they retreat into silence? Understanding how partners handled these emotions can lead to more effective strategies moving forward. For many, acknowledging jealousy as a natural response rather than a failure can shift the narrative, enabling partners to approach these feelings with empathy and understanding rather than fear or shame.

The dynamics of raising children in polyamorous families also warrant careful reflection. Couples may explore how their parenting styles and values have evolved through their polyamorous journey. Discussions around discipline, emotional support, and the importance of transparency with children about family structures can provide clarity. By reflecting on their parenting experiences, partners can identify areas that align with their values as a family and address any inconsistencies that may arise. They can also consider how their relationships with one another influence their children's understanding of love, commitment, and family.

Finally, personal growth and self-discovery are integral to the polyamorous experience. As couples reflect on their journey, they may recognize how their relationships have catalyzed personal development. Each partner's exploration of their identity, desires, and boundaries can lead to profound insights about themselves and their roles within the marriage. This journey is not just about nurturing connections with multiple partners but also about fostering individual growth that enriches the primary relationship. By sharing these reflections, couples can create a supportive environment that values both individuality and togetherness, ultimately strengthening the fabric of their polyamorous marriage.

Embracing the Future of Polyamorous Relationships

Embracing the future of polyamorous relationships requires a commitment to open communication, emotional intelligence, and an understanding of the unique dynamics that come with non-monogamous partnerships. As society continues to evolve, so too do the frameworks through which we view love, commitment, and family structures. In polyamorous marriages, partners often find themselves navigating a complex landscape of emotions, relationships, and societal expectations. By adopting effective communication strategies, couples can create a foundation that not only supports their romantic connections but also fosters personal growth and resilience.

One of the most significant challenges faced by those in polyamorous marriages is managing feelings of jealousy and insecurity. These emotions can arise from various sources, including fear of abandonment, comparison to other partners, or a perceived lack of attention from a primary partner. To embrace the future of polyamorous relationships, couples must actively engage in conversations that address these feelings head-on. Techniques such as "feelings check-ins" and "root cause exploration" can provide partners with the opportunity to express their insecurities in a safe space, ultimately leading to deeper understanding and emotional intimacy. By validating each other's feelings and working collaboratively to address insecurities, couples can cultivate a more secure and trusting environment.

Raising children in polyamorous families introduces another layer of complexity, highlighting the need for clear communication and shared values among all adults involved. It is essential for parents to discuss their parenting philosophies, boundaries, and the roles that each partner will play in the children's lives. Open discussions about family dynamics can help children feel secure and supported, regardless of the number of adults involved in their upbringing. By modeling healthy communication and emotional expression, polyamorous parents can instill in their children a sense of acceptance and understanding of diverse family structures, preparing them to navigate their own relationships in an increasingly interconnected world.

Support systems play a crucial role in the success of polyamorous marriages. Establishing a network of like-minded individuals can provide couples with resources, encouragement, and the reassurance that they are not alone in their journey. This support can come in various forms, including polyamory-focused meetups, online communities, and workshops that emphasize communication and relationship skills. By seeking out these networks, couples can share experiences, gain insights from others who have faced similar challenges, and forge connections that reinforce their commitment to a polyamorous lifestyle. Building a strong support system enhances resilience and provides a safety net during difficult times.

Ultimately, embracing the future of polyamorous relationships involves a commitment to personal growth and self-discovery. Engaging in multiple relationships can serve as a catalyst for individuals to explore their desires, boundaries, and emotional needs. Encouraging each partner to pursue their interests and passions not only enriches their personal lives but also strengthens the marriage as a whole. By nurturing a culture of self-exploration within the framework of polyamory, couples can foster deeper connections and a more profound understanding of themselves and each other. In doing so, they pave the way for a future where love is abundant, multifaceted, and fulfilling.

Final Thoughts on Communication and Connection

Effective communication forms the bedrock of any successful relationship, but it takes on even greater significance in polyamorous marriages. With multiple partners involved, the potential for misunderstandings and misinterpretations increases. Couples must prioritize open dialogue, ensuring that all voices are heard and respected. This entails not just talking but also actively listening. By fostering an environment where partners can express their thoughts, feelings, and concerns without fear of judgment, couples can build deeper connections and navigate the complexities of their relationships more seamlessly.

Jealousy and insecurity are common challenges in polyamorous dynamics, often arising from perceived threats or the fear of losing a partner's affection. To combat these feelings, couples should engage in regular check-ins centered around emotional states and relationship dynamics. Encouraging transparency about insecurities allows partners to provide reassurance and support, transforming moments of vulnerability into opportunities for intimacy. Effective communication strategies, such as using "I" statements and focusing on feelings rather than accusations, can help partners express their concerns without escalating tensions.

For couples raising children within a polyamorous framework, the importance of communication cannot be overstated. Parents must navigate the complexities of co-parenting while also addressing the unique challenges that arise from their relationship structure. Establishing clear communication channels among all adults involved is essential for creating a stable and supportive environment for children. Regular family meetings can help ensure that everyone is on the same page about parenting philosophies, schedules, and the emotional needs of the children. This collective approach not only strengthens the family unit but also models healthy communication for the next generation.

Building a robust support system is crucial for couples in polyamorous marriages. This can include friends, family, or community groups that understand and accept their relationship dynamics. Open communication about the need for support is vital; partners should feel empowered to reach out for help when necessary. Sharing experiences and challenges with others who have similar lifestyles can provide new insights and coping strategies. This network serves as an emotional buffer, helping couples to feel less isolated and more understood in their unique journeys.

Lastly, polyamorous marriages offer a unique opportunity for personal growth and self-discovery. As partners navigate their relationships, they often uncover new aspects of themselves that may have remained dormant within a monogamous framework. Encouraging open dialogue about individual aspirations, fears, and desires fosters an environment where partners can grow together while also supporting each other's personal journeys. By embracing this dual focus on communication and connection, couples can create a thriving polyamorous marriage that honors both their collective and individual needs.